INTESTINAL SURGERY RECOVERY DIET

Complete Guide Unlocking The Secrets Of
Nutrition To Rapid Healing After Surgery
Success, Nourishing Meal Plans, Recipes, Tips
For Optimal Health Wellness)

DR. ALLAN FREDA

Contents

CHAPTER 1..5

HOW TO RECOVER FROM INTESTINAL SURGERY.......5

CHAPTER 2..19

GETTING READY FOR RECOVERY 19

CHAPTER 3 25

THE BUILDING BLOCKS OF A HEALING DIET 25

CHAPTER 4 36

PLANNING MEALS FOR OPTIMAL HEALTH................36

CHAPTER 5 40

DEALING WITH DIGESTIVE PROBLEMS.......................40

CHAPTER 7 51

MINDFUL EATING TO GET BETTER 51

CHAPTER 8 55

BEYOND THE PLATE: HOLISTIC PRACTICES FOR RECOVERY 55

CHAPTER 9..60

RECIPES FOR HEALING...60

CHAPTER 10..67

KEEPS YOUR HEALTH IN THE LONG TERM 67

CONCLUSION 71

1. How to Know How Important Food Is for Healing After Having GI Surgery:

o An explanation of how a good diet helps the body heal, lowers the risk of complications and improves long-term health.

o An overview of important chemicals and how they help the body heal.

2. Advice and tips from experts:

o Help from nutritionists, dietitians, and medical workers who specialize in helping people recover from surgery.

Strategies that have been shown to work for dealing with nutritional problems like digestive issues and problems absorbing nutrients.

3. Meal plans and recipes that heal:

o Nutrient-dense recipes that are meant to help with recovery and healing.

o Well-balanced meal plans that are adapted to different stages of healing to make sure that people get enough food while minimizing pain.

4. Long-Term Plans for Health:

o Eating habits that will last so that intestinal health is supported after the recovery time is over.

Tips on how to keep up healthy eating and living habits for general well-being.

Proven Tip: Eat foods that reduce inflammation, like nuts, berries, leafy veggies, and fatty fish, while you're healing. These foods help lower swelling, speed up the healing process, and support tissue repair.

CHAPTER 1
HOW TO RECOVER FROM INTESTINAL SURGERY

When you have intestine surgery, a doctor will fix several problems with your digestive system.

After surgery, you will need to carefully follow a special diet plan to help your body heal and get better as quickly as possible. This detailed guide goes into great detail about how to eat after surgery, showing how important food choices are for helping people heal and stay healthy in the long run after having surgery on their intestines.

A Look at Surgery on the Intestines

Intestinal surgery includes a wide range of treatments used to treat problems with the digestive system, which includes the large and small intestines. Whether it's because of inflammatory bowel diseases (IBD) like Crohn's disease or ulcerative colitis, gastrointestinal cancers, diverticulitis, or other GI problems, these surgeries are meant to ease symptoms, fix structural problems, or get rid of diseased tissue. The level of difficulty of a procedure can range from slightly invasive laparoscopic surgeries to open surgeries that remove and rebuild a lot of tissue. Which surgical method is used depends on things like the type and severity of the underlying condition, the patient's general health, and the way the body is built?

Common Procedures and What They Mean

Several common surgeries are done on the intestines to treat a wide range of digestive problems. Each has its effects on healing after surgery. For diseases like colon cancer, ulcerative colitis, or familial adenomatous polyposis (FAP), a colectomy may be necessary.

This procedure involves removing part or all of the colon. In serious cases of inflammatory bowel disease, ileal pouch-anal anastomosis (IPAA) surgery may be done to replace the colon and rectum with a reservoir from the small intestine. This keeps the person's continence. Bowel resections may be needed to remove parts of the diseased gut that are affected by Crohn's disease, intestinal obstructions, or perforations.

During ostomy surgeries, like colostomy and ileostomy, a stoma is made to redirect feces, which can help with conditions like colorectal cancer, diverticulitis, or injuries. For each treatment, there are different challenges and things to think about when it comes to postoperative care, such as making changes to your diet to help you heal, avoid complications, and get the best results.

How Important Food Is for Recovery

Nutrition is very important for healing after surgery on the intestines because it has a big impact on how well the wounds heal, how well the immune system works, how well the intestines move, and general health.

To meet the higher metabolic needs that come with healing tissues, boosting the immune system, and using more energy after surgery, it is important to get enough calories. Getting the right nutrition before and after surgery can lower the chance of problems like infection, wound dehiscence, malnutrition, and taking longer to recover. Additionally, some digestive problems may need special dietary changes to help ease symptoms, lower inflammation, and speed up the healing process in the intestines. Surgeons, dietitians, and other healthcare workers must work together to create individualized nutrition plans that meet the specific needs of patients having surgery on their intestines.

A complete guide to the best diet for people who have just had surgery, with healing recipes, meal plans, and expert advice for long-term health.

Managing your diet after surgery can be hard. You need a multifaceted approach that includes evidence-based dietary guidelines, useful meal-planning tools, and expert advice on what your body needs during the recovery time. This complete guide is meant to give people who have just been diagnosed with gastrointestinal disorders and need surgery the information and tools they need to make the best choices about what they eat after surgery to help them heal, recover, and stay healthy in the long run.

Understanding What to Eat After Surgery on the Digestive System

When someone has surgery on their intestines, what they eat becomes very important for helping them recover, healing, and lowering their risk of health problems after the surgery.

People may have changes in how their digestive system works, how well they absorb nutrients, and how well they can handle certain foods. Because of this, they may need to make slow changes to their diets that are based on their specific needs and the results of their surgery.

Improving nutrient intake, controlling digestive symptoms, encouraging regular bowel movements, and avoiding nutritional deficiencies are some of the most important things to think about when planning your diet after surgery on your intestines. It's important for healthcare professionals like surgeons, dietitians, and nutritionists to work together to come up with personalized meal plans that meet the unique needs and problems that come up after surgery.

Getting the Most Nutrients

Getting enough nutrients is important for helping tissues heal, the immune system work, and general recovery after surgery on the intestines. Protein-rich foods are very important for wound healing and tissue regeneration because they contain the vital amino acids that cells need to make collagen and heal themselves. Adding lean protein sources like chicken, fish, tofu, beans, and dairy products to your diet can help you meet your higher protein needs after surgery. Also, getting enough micronutrients, like vitamins and minerals, is important for keeping your immune system healthy, helping tissues heal, and avoiding nutritional deficits. You can get a lot of important vitamins and minerals from fresh fruits, veggies, whole grains, nuts, and seeds. These vitamins and minerals help your body heal wounds, fight free radicals, and keep your bones healthy. Focusing on a healthy, well-balanced diet full of nutrient-dense foods can help you get the most nutrients and speed up your healing after surgery on your intestines.

Taking Care of Problems in the Gut

Postoperative gastrointestinal symptoms like stomach pain, bloating, gas, diarrhea, or constipation can make it hard to stick to a diet and absorb nutrients. To ease symptoms and improve gastrointestinal comfort, specific dietary changes may be needed. Gradually returning to solid foods after surgery and avoiding eating too many high-fat, high-fiber, or gas-causing foods can help keep stomach problems to a minimum and make oral intake easier.

Soluble fiber sources like oats, applesauce, bananas, and steamed veggies can help keep your bowels regular and ease constipation after surgery without making your stomach problems worse. Foods that are high in probiotics, like yogurt, kefir, and fermented veggies, may also help restore the balance of microbiota in the gut and improve digestive function after surgery. Keeping an eye on how sensitive each person is to certain foods and making changes to their diet as needed can help them feel better and get all the nutrients they need while they are recovering.

Getting Bowels to Move Regularly

Having regular bowel movements is important to avoid problems like constipation, fecal impaction, or bowel obstruction after surgery, which can hurt the patient's health and the success of the surgery. Adequate fluid intake, food fiber, and physical activity are all important for keeping bowel movements regular and avoiding problems with gastrointestinal motility after surgery on the intestines. Regularly drinking water, herbal drinks, clear broths, and other fluids high in electrolytes can help keep you from becoming dehydrated and soften your stools, making them easier to pass and relieving constipation.

Adding more fiber to your diet slowly from foods like whole grains, fruits, veggies, and legumes can help your colon move, make stools bulkier, and keep them that way without making your digestive problems worse.

As well, doing light exercises like walking or easy stretching can help stimulate peristalsis, which can improve bowel motility and ease gastrointestinal pain after surgery. Having a normal bowel routine and keeping an eye on your bowel habits can help you spot problems early and take the right steps to improve your bowel function after surgery.

People who have had intestinal surgery may be more likely to not get enough nutrients because of changes in their gastrointestinal anatomy, problems absorbing nutrients, or dietary limits put in place after surgery.

Regular checks of body measures, biochemical markers, and food intake can help find and fix any nutritional problems quickly by showing how well someone is doing in terms of nutrition.

Vitamin, mineral, or micronutrient supplements may be needed if a person isn't getting enough of certain nutrients from their food, has a malabsorption disease, or has had surgery and isn't getting enough of certain nutrients.

Dietitians, doctors, and other health care professionals need to work together to come up with individualized supplementation plans for people having intestinal surgery that are specific to their needs and situations.

Focusing on a variety of nutrient-dense foods and keeping an eye on your nutritional state regularly can help lower the risk of nutritional deficiencies, speed up recovery, and promote long-term health after intestinal surgery.

Planning and practically making meals can help people who are healing from intestinal surgery follow the diet suggestions made by their surgeons, make sure they get enough nutrients and enjoy eating more.

Adding different tastes, textures, and nutrient-dense foods to your meals can make them more enjoyable, help you feel full, and make you happier with your diet without lowering the nutritional value.

Batch cooking and food prepping ahead of time can make it easier to make meals, free up time, and make sure that you have access to healthy meals while you are recovering from surgery. Getting family, carers, or support networks involved in planning and making meals can also help build social support, reduce stress, and give you a sense of calm while you're recovering.

Adding healing recipes with nutrient-dense foods, herbs, and spices known for their anti-inflammatory, antioxidant, or digestive qualities can make the diet after surgery more interesting and helpful.

Getting help from doctors, dietitians, or chefs can be very helpful when planning meals, making changes to recipes, and coming up with dietary plans that fit your tastes, dietary limits, and nutritional needs after intestinal surgery.

Tips from experts for long-term health

Long-term health after surgery on the intestines depends on making changes to your diet, lifestyle, and self-care habits that will last. These changes should improve your general quality of life, keep your intestines healthy, and stop diseases from coming back.

Managing your stress, getting enough exercise, and following good sleep habits can all help your immune system work better, lower inflammation, and speed up your recovery after surgery.

Focusing on nutrient-dense foods, mindful eating, and amount control can help you have a good relationship with food, feel full, and avoid gaining or losing too much weight after intestinal surgery.

Keeping an eye on your symptoms, going to your follow-up visits, and talking to your healthcare providers regularly can help you find complications early, get help right away, and get support as you recover from surgery.

People who are dealing with the difficulties of living with gastrointestinal disorders after surgery can get emotional support, useful information, and a sense of empowerment from joining peer support groups, educational tools, or counseling services. Building resilience, self-compassion, and adaptive coping skills can help people accept their postoperative journey, deal with challenges, and take a whole-person approach to their long-term health and quality of life after intestinal surgery.

CHAPTER 2
GETTING READY FOR RECOVERY

For the best healing after surgery on the intestines, whether it's for inflammatory bowel disease, diverticulitis, or cancer, it's important to plan.

The post-surgery diet is an important part of this planning because it helps with healing, managing symptoms, and getting the digestive system back to normal. Before getting into the details of an intestinal surgery recovery diet, it's important to talk about what people can do ahead of time to make the recovery process go more smoothly.

Dietary Things to Think About Before Surgery

People who are going to have surgery on their intestines should pay close attention to what they eat before the operation. It is very important to follow any pre-operative dietary advice given by a medical worker.

Nonetheless, there are a few general considerations.

First, making sure you get enough food and water is important for your general health and ability to recover from surgery.

This could mean eating a healthy, well-balanced meal full of fruits, vegetables, whole grains, lean proteins, and healthy fats. Also, drinking a lot of water is important to stay refreshed so that your body can keep working properly and help the healing process.

In some cases, doctors may tell patients to make certain changes to their diets in the days before surgery. People with inflammatory bowel disease, for example, may be told to follow a low-residue diet to cut down on bowel movements and lower the risk of problems during surgery.

In the same way, people who have certain food allergies or intolerances should stay away from foods that make them sick before or after surgery.

A person who have had surgery on their intestines often starts to feel better at home, where they can create a supportive setting that helps them heal. This includes things like making sure they are physically comfortable, giving them mental support, and helping them with their daily tasks. Family members or carers can be very helpful by offering support, helping with chores around the house, and making sure that medicine is taken as prescribed.

When it comes to dietary support, it's helpful to think ahead and stock up on healthy foods that are in line with the diet suggestions after surgery. Making an eating area that is comfy and free of distractions can also help you eat more mindfully and digest food better. Supporting someone emotionally is also very important since surgery can be upsetting. Patients should be able to talk about their feelings and wants with the people who are helping them, like friends, family, or healthcare professionals.

One way to make sure you heal quickly after surgery on your intestines is to make sure your kitchen is full of healthy foods that are easy on the digestive system. This needs careful planning and shopping for foods that meet the nutrition needs set by healthcare professionals.

First and foremost, it's important to choose foods that are easy to digest and don't hurt the stomach or bowels. This includes cooked veggies like potatoes, carrots, and squash, lean proteins like chicken, turkey, and fish, and grains that are easy to digest like white rice, oatmeal, and quinoa.

Adding foods that are high in vitamins, minerals, and antioxidants can also help the body heal and improve health in general.

When preparing the kitchen for recovery after surgery, it's also important to think about any dietary needs or limits.

 For instance, people who can't handle lactose may choose dairy-free options, and people who can't handle gluten should choose grains and goods that don't contain gluten.

Carefully reading food labels and choosing whole, slightly processed foods can help you stay away from possible triggers and keep your digestive system healthy.

Along with solid foods, it's important to have a lot of drinks that will keep you hydrated, like water, herbal teas, and drinks that are high in electrolytes. Staying hydrated is important for keeping your body working, avoiding dehydration, and healing properly after surgery.

Overall, having a range of healthy, easily digestible foods and drinks in your kitchen can help you recover quickly and well from intestinal surgery.

Patients can speed up their recovery and set themselves up for long-term health by choosing foods that are high in nutrients and taking their individual nutritional needs into account.

CHAPTER 3
THE BUILDING BLOCKS OF A HEALING DIET

Before getting into the details of a diet for recovery after surgery, it's important to understand the basic ideas that make it work. You can't just eat any food on a healing diet; you have to choose foods that are high in nutrients and help the body's natural mending processes. In this part, we'll talk about how to stay hydrated, eat foods that are high in nutrients, and make sure that your macronutrients (proteins, carbs, and fats) are balanced for the best recovery.

Foods High in Nutrients for Healing

Including foods that are high in nutrients is an important part of a healthy diet. There are a lot of vitamins, minerals, antioxidants, and other bioactive substances in these foods that are important for cell repair and regeneration. Many different kinds of fruits, veggies, lean proteins, whole grains, and healthy fats are important for making sure the body gets all the nutrients it needs to heal.

Because they are high in vitamins, minerals, and phytonutrients, fruits and veggies are especially good for you. Antioxidants in these plant-based foods help lower inflammation and protect against oxidative stress. Both of these are very important for helping the body heal and keep the immune system working well while you're recovering.

Fruits and veggies also contain dietary fiber, which helps the digestive system and improves gut health, which is an important part of overall health, especially after surgery on the intestines.

Lean proteins are also an important part of a healing diet because they give your body the building blocks it needs to heal tissues and build muscles. High-quality protein can be found in foods like chicken, fish, tofu, lentils, and low-fat dairy products.

These foods don't have a lot of saturated fat, which can make inflammation worse and slow down the healing process. Including protein-rich foods at every meal can help you feel full, keep your blood sugar stable, and help your body heal.

Whole grains are a good source of complex carbohydrates, which give your body long-lasting energy to help it heal. Whole grains release glucose slowly, which helps keep energy levels steady throughout the day. This is different from refined carbs, which are broken down quickly and can cause blood sugar to rise. Whole grains are also a good addition to any diet after surgery because they contain fiber, vitamins, and minerals that are good for your health and well-being as a whole.

Healthy fats are very important for keeping cells working, making hormones, and controlling inflammation.

Unsaturated fats found in avocados, nuts, seeds, and olive oil are good for your heart and help lower inflammation, which is especially helpful while you're healing. Omega-3 fatty acids, which can be found in flaxseeds and fatty fish like salmon, have been shown to reduce inflammation and may help the body heal after surgery.

When planning a diet for recovery after surgery, focusing on nutrient-rich foods is important because they give the body the nutrients it needs to heal and stay healthy. There are many vitamins, minerals, antioxidants, and other bioactive compounds in fruits, veggies, lean proteins, whole grains, and healthy fats that help the body heal by reducing inflammation, repairing tissues, and supporting immune function.

How to Stay Hydrated

Another important part of a healing diet is staying hydrated. Drinking enough water is needed for many bodily processes, such as digestion, nutrient absorption, circulation, and getting rid of toxins. Dehydration can make these processes less efficient and make it harder for the body to recover from surgery. So, keeping your body at the right level of hydration is very important for healing and general health.

As the main way to stay hydrated, you should drink water throughout the day to keep from becoming dehydrated. Besides regular water, you can also drink herbal teas, broths, and fruit juices that have been diluted. But it's important to stay away from sugary and caffeinated drinks in large amounts during the recovery time because they can dehydrate you and make inflammation and pain worse.

Checking the color and frequency of your pee can tell you a lot about how well you're hydrated. If your urine is clear or pale yellow, it means you're getting enough water. If your urine is dark yellow or amber, it could mean you're dehydrated and need to drink more water.

People who have recently had surgery should try to drink enough water to keep their pee light and avoid getting thirsty since thirst is often a sign of being dehydrated.

Extra water may be needed in some situations, especially if the person is losing a lot of fluids because of things like heat, vomiting, diarrhea, or sweating a lot. Oral rehydration solutions with electrolytes like sodium, potassium, and chloride can help more than water alone to recover the balance of fluids and electrolytes in this case.

You can easily find these solutions at pharmacies. They can be especially helpful for people healing from intestinal surgery who may lose fluids or have electrolyte imbalances.

Keep in mind that everyone's fluid needs are different, depending on their age, body weight, amount of activity, the weather, and their overall health.

To stay properly hydrated during the recovery period, it is important to pay attention to your body's thirst signals and change how much water you drink appropriately. Prioritizing staying hydrated and drinking a range of fluids throughout the day can help the body heal and speed up the recovery process after intestinal surgery.

Proteins, carbohydrates, and fats need to be balanced.

In addition to eating nutrient-dense foods and staying hydrated, it is important to get the right amount of macronutrients (proteins, carbohydrates, and fats) to help with recovery and improve general health after intestinal surgery. Every macronutrient is important for different parts of mending and recovery and has its effect on the body's physiology.

Proteins are important for repairing and rebuilding cells that have been damaged during surgery, which is why they are often called the body's building blocks. Wound healing, muscle regeneration, and immune system performance need to get enough protein. People who have recently had surgery should try to eat protein-rich foods with every meal and snack to help their bodies heal and keep their muscles from losing mass.

Lean meats, chicken, fish, eggs, dairy products, legumes, tofu, and tempeh are all good sources of high-quality protein. Essential amino acids are the building blocks of protein. The body can't make them on its own, so it needs to get them from food. Getting protein from a range of sources helps the body get all the amino acids it needs to repair tissues and keep muscle mass while it recovers.

Carbohydrates are the body's main source of energy and are needed to power cellular processes, keep you active, and replace glycogen stores that were lost during surgery and healing.

However, not all carbohydrates are the same. To keep your blood sugar levels stable and your energy up all day, it's important to choose complex carbohydrates over refined carbohydrates.

These are foods like whole grains, fruits, veggies, and legumes.

Complex carbs are good for your health because they have fiber, vitamins, and minerals. Refined carbohydrates, on the other hand, are high in empty calories and may make inflammation and insulin resistance worse. People can meet their energy needs, feel full, and help their bodies heal better after surgery by putting complex carbs at the top of their food list.

When it comes to supporting cell activity, hormone production, and nutrient absorption, fats are another important macronutrient. Fats have a bad reputation in the past, but a new study shows that eating healthy fats like those in avocados, nuts, seeds, olive oil, and fatty fish can help your health in many ways, like lowering inflammation and keeping your heart healthy.

Researchers have looked into omega-3 fatty acids, in particular, to see if they can help with inflammation and possibly speed up mending and lower the risk of complications after surgery. Some foods that are high in omega-3 fatty acids are salmon, mackerel, sardines, flaxseeds, and walnuts. These foods can help the body recover from surgery and improve general health during this time.

getting the right number of macronutrients (proteins, carbs, and fats) is important for helping the body recover from intestinal surgery and staying healthy in the long run. Focusing on protein-rich foods can help fix damaged tissues and build new muscles. On the other hand, choosing complex carbohydrates gives you long-lasting energy and important nutrients. Adding healthy fats to your diet helps cells work better and lowers inflammation, which makes it easier for your body to heal and recover. Focusing on a balanced intake of macronutrients can help people get the most out of their diet after surgery, which will help them recover quickly and stay healthy in the long run.

CHAPTER 4
PLANNING MEALS FOR OPTIMAL HEALTH

Making Snacks and Healing Foods:

Making healthy meals and snacks for people who have had surgery on their intestines is important for helping their bodies heal and improving their general health. These meals should be carefully planned to make sure they provide the right calories, help digestion, and ease pain.

Eating foods that are high in fiber, vitamins, minerals, and protein can help your body heal and fight off illness. Focusing on foods that are easy to digest, like lean proteins, cooked veggies, whole grains, and fruits, can help reduce stomach problems and speed up the healing process. Adding healing plants and spices like garlic, ginger, and turmeric can also help reduce inflammation and kill germs, which makes the healing process even stronger.

Snacks like smoothies, yogurt with fruit, boiled eggs, or nut butter on whole-grain toast are high in nutrients and easy to stomach. They give you long-lasting energy and help your body heal properly.

It is important to make sample meal plans that are suited to different stages of healing to make sure that people get enough food while also taking into account their changing dietary needs and tolerances. In the first few days after surgery, when the digestive system is at its weakest, meals should consist of drinks and foods that are easy to digest to keep the person from feeling sick or in pain. Some examples of this are clear broths, herbal teas, gelatin, and small amounts of mashed fruits and veggies. As your body gets stronger and your tolerance grows, slowly adding soft, low-fiber foods like scrambled eggs, cooked cereals, steamed veggies, and lean meats can help you get the nutrients you need while reducing stress on your digestive system. Lastly, switching to a regular diet that includes lots of fruits and vegetables, lean proteins, and healthy fats can help your body heal and stay healthy in the long run. To speed up recovery and help people stick to their post-surgery diet, it's important to change portion sizes and meal times based on each person's needs and tastes.

Adding different tastes and textures:

Adding variety and flavor to meals after surgery is important for making them more enjoyable and helping people stick to their healing diet. At first, dietary restrictions may make it hard to choose what to eat, but trying out different cooking methods, seasonings, and combinations of ingredients can help you make meals that are both tasty and filling. Experimenting with different herbs, spices, and condiments can make bland foods taste better, making them more fun to eat.

Adding different colors and textures to foods can also stimulate the senses and make people hungrier, which can encourage them to eat a wider range of nutrients. Adding a variety of umami, sweet, savory, sour, and savory flavors can make the meal more enjoyable and help you feel full. Involving the person in planning and making their meals can also give them the power to make healthier choices and make them feel more involved in their healing. By focusing on flavor and variety, meals after surgery can be both healthy and fun, helping with the best healing and long-term health.

CHAPTER 5
DEALING WITH DIGESTIVE PROBLEMS

Digestive problems can be a big problem for people who are having surgery on their intestines and then recovering. Not only does the operating site have to heal physically, but digestion also has to get back to normal after surgery on the intestines.

This complete guide tries to give you information on how to deal with digestive problems after surgery, with a focus on ways to ease pain, improve digestive function, and promote long-term health through healthy eating.

How to Deal with Digestive Pain

People who have had surgery on their intestines often have stomach problems while their bodies get used to the changes in their structure and function. Symptoms like bloating, gas, constipation, diarrhea, and abdominal pain can happen for many reasons, such as the effects of anesthesia, changes in food, and surgery-related injuries. Taking care of digestive pain requires a multifaceted method that treats the underlying causes as well as the symptoms.

Diet changes are one of the most important things to think about when you have stomach problems. At first, patients may be given a clear liquid diet to rest their digestive system.

As they can handle it, they can slowly switch to a more varied diet.

During the recovery time, staying away from foods that are known to make symptoms worse, like those that are spicy, greasy, or high in fiber, can help ease the pain. Eating smaller meals more often and eating your food can also make your digestive system work better and lessen the effects of bloating and gas.

Adding gentle exercises like walking to your daily routine can help your bowels move more easily and relieve constipation.

However, it is important to talk to a doctor or nurse before doing any physical action after surgery to make sure it is safe and right for you.

Also, staying hydrated by drinking lots of fluids, usually water, can help soften stools and keep you from becoming dehydrated, both of which are important for keeping your digestive system working well.

During the recovery time after surgery, some foods can help ease digestive problems and speed up the healing process. Choose foods that are easy to digest and low in fat and fiber to make your digestive system's job easier and reduce pain. Some examples are

1. Clear fluids: Herbal teas, clear soups, broths, and electrolyte-rich drinks can keep you hydrated and

give you the nutrients you need without putting too much stress on your digestive system.

2. Soft, cooked vegetables: Carrots, squash, and zucchini, which can be steamed or boiled, are easy on the stomach and give you the vitamins and minerals you need to heal.

3. Lean protein sources: Chicken breasts without skin, fish, tofu, and eggs are all good sources of protein that are less likely to upset your stomach than fatty or highly processed meats.

4. Low-fiber carbs: White rice, muesli, and refined grains are easier to digest than whole grains.

They can give you energy without making your digestive problems worse.

5. Fermented foods: Probiotics found in yogurt, kefir, and fermented greens are good for your gut health and may help keep digestion in check.

But different people may not be able to handle the same foods.

It is important to pay attention to your body's signs and stay away from foods that make you feel bad or make your symptoms worse.

Taking steps to improve digestive function can help with long-term recovery and wellness, in addition to handling immediate post-surgery symptoms.

Eating a healthy, well-balanced diet full of fruits, veggies, whole grains, lean proteins, and healthy fats can give you the nutrients you need and help your digestive health as a whole.

Fiber-rich foods, like fruits, veggies, legumes, and whole grains, help keep your bowel movements regular and keep you from getting constipated if you eat them slowly and drink enough water.

Adding probiotic-rich foods or supplements to your diet can also help reset the balance of good bacteria in your gut, which is important for healthy digestion and immune function. Probiotics are found in fermented foods like cabbage, kimchi, yogurt, and kefir.

They can also be taken as a supplement. Nevertheless, it is suggested that you talk to your doctor before beginning any new vitamins, especially after surgery.

Being aware of your eating habits, like taking your time to chew each bite fully and slowly, not eating too much, and noticing when you're hungry or full, can help your stomach work better and keep you from feeling uncomfortable. Manage stress through deep breathing, meditation, or gentle yoga. These methods can also help the digestive system by lowering cortisol levels and putting the body into a state of relaxation.

dealing with digestive problems after surgery on the intestines requires a multifaceted approach that includes changing the diet, treating symptoms, and planning ways to improve digestive function in the long run. A balanced diet, gentle physical activity, and learning how to deal with stress are all things that people can do to help their recovery and improve their general health. Talking to doctors and nurses, like surgeons, dietitians, and gastroenterologists, can give people personalised advice and help during their recovery, making sure they have the best outcomes possible after intestinal surgery.

IMPROVED IMMUNE SUPPORT IN CHAPTER 6

The body goes through a big stress response after having surgery on the intestines, so it's important to support the immune system for the best healing. At this point, you need to take a broad look at your diet and habits to help your immune system work better and speed up the healing process. Adding immune-boosting foods and nutrients, antioxidants for healing, and thinking about different living factors that affect immune health are all ways to improve immune support after surgery.

Good for your immune system foods and nutrients

Diet is one of the most important things that can help your immune system after treatment of your intestines. It is important to choose foods that are high in necessary nutrients that your immune system needs to work well. Citrus fruits, cherries, and bell peppers all have a lot of vitamin C, which helps make collagen and improves the function of immune cells. Vitamin E, which can be found in nuts, seeds, and leafy veggies, also protects cells from damage as an antioxidant. Zinc, which can be found in meat, shellfish, beans, and nuts, helps immune cells work and wounds heal, which is very important during the recovery phase. Fish, eggs, lean meats, and vegetables are all high in protein. Protein-rich foods help immune cells and tissues heal. Adding probiotic-rich foods like yogurt, kefir, and fermented veggies to your diet can also help keep your gut microbiome healthy, which is important for your immune system. Also, omega-3 fatty acids found in fatty fish, flaxseeds, and peanuts can help keep your immune system healthy by reducing inflammation. People who have had intestinal surgery can boost their immune systems by making sure they eat a lot of these immunity-boosting nutrients.

Using antioxidants to help with healing

Antioxidants are very important for mending after surgery because they reduce oxidative stress and swelling. Adding a range of antioxidant-rich foods to the recovery diet can help the body heal faster and avoid problems. Berry, cherry, and grapefruits, as well as spinach, kale, and broccoli vegetables, are great places to get antioxidants like vitamin C, vitamin E, and different phytonutrients.

These chemicals get rid of the free radicals that are made during surgery and help the tissue heal. Herbs and spices like garlic, ginger, and turmeric are also very good at fighting inflammation and free radicals, which helps the body heal even more. Herbal teas with antioxidants can also be helpful adds to a diet after surgery because they help the immune system and keep you hydrated at the same time. People who have had intestinal surgery can speed up the mending process and lower their risk of complications by eating and drinking a variety of antioxidant-rich foods and drinks.

In addition to what you eat, how you live your life has a big effect on how well your immune system works after intestine surgery. Getting enough sleep is very important because it helps defense cells work and tissues heal. Setting a regular sleep routine and making your bedroom a good place to sleep can help you get the rest you need to heal properly.

Managing stress is also very important because long-term worry can weaken the immune system and make it harder to heal. Adding stress-relieving activities like focused meditation, deep breathing exercises, or gentle yoga can help the immune system deal with stress better.

Regular physical exercise, based on each person's abilities after surgery, not only improves blood flow and oxygenation to tissues but also makes the immune system work better. It's important to talk to medical professionals to figure out the right amount of activity and exercises for each person based on their condition and recovery progress.

Also, good hygiene, like washing your hands often and getting vaccinated as suggested, helps keep you from getting infections that could weaken your immune system while you're recovering.

By addressing these lifestyle factors along with dietary concerns, people can strengthen their immune systems and speed up the healing process after surgery on the intestines.

CHAPTER 7
MINDFUL EATING TO GET BETTER

It takes a lot of work to recover from surgery on the intestines, and what you eat is a very important part of that. During this time of healing, practicing mindful eating can make it much easier for the body to heal and get stronger. Being fully present and aware of the food you eat, how it makes you feel, and how it affects your body is what mindfulness means when you eat. It stresses the link between the mind and body, which helps people have a better relationship with food and improves their general health.

Why mindfulness is important for healing

Being mindful about what you eat is especially important after treatment on your intestines for several reasons. First, it tells people to pay attention to their bodies and understand when they are hungry or full, which may be different after surgery. Being aware of this can help you avoid either overeating or undereating, which can slow down the repair process. Mindful eating also helps the body handle food better and absorb nutrients better because it lets the body fully participate in the eating process. It also lowers stress and anxiety about food, which can happen a lot during recovery, and it improves mental and emotional health, both of which are important for healing generally.

Ways to Eat More Mindfully

There are several ways that people can practice mindful eating while they are recovering from surgery on their intestines. Mindful breathing is one of these techniques. To center yourself and become more aware of the present moment, take deep breaths before and during meals.

Another good tip is to chew your food slowly and enjoy every bite. This helps your body digest food better and enjoy flavors more.

Engaging all the senses by noticing how food feels, smells, and looks can also make the experience of mindful eating better. Mindful eating also means avoiding screens like TVs and electronics during meals so that you can fully focus on the act of eating and how it affects your body.

Developing a Healthy Connection with Food

It can be hard to get back to normal after surgery on your intestines, and having a healthy relationship with food is important for long-term health. Mindful eating can help people have a better relationship with food by teaching them to be kind to themselves and not judge others.

Mindful eating tells people not to label foods as "good" or "bad," but to look at them with interest and an open mind, knowing that all foods can be part of a healthy diet. It also makes you feel grateful for the food that feeds you and gives you control over the food you eat. Mindfulness can help people develop a healthy relationship with food, which can help them on their way to recovery and help them form habits that are good for their general health and well-being.

 practicing mindful eating while recovering from surgery on the intestines can speed up the healing process and improve health in the long run. People can help their bodies heal and build a healthy relationship with food by focusing on being aware, making choices, and being kind to themselves when they eat.

Mindful breathing, slow chewing, and limiting distractions are some ways that people can fully enjoy eating and get the most nutrients out of their food. Practicing awareness while eating not only helps the body heal but also improves mental and emotional health, which is an important part of a whole-person approach to recovery and long-term health.

CHAPTER 8
BEYOND THE PLATE: HOLISTIC PRACTICES FOR RECOVERY

When trying to get better after surgery on the intestines, focusing only on changes to the diet could mean missing out on the whole-person method that is needed for full recovery. Rather than just making changes to your diet, holistic recovery practices include a wide range of methods meant to improve your general health, assist with physical recovery, and strengthen your emotional strength. This detailed guide covers three important parts of total recovery: Including Safely Moving and Working Out, Dealing with Stress, and Making Connections with Helpful People.

Physical exercise is very important for recovery after surgery because it improves mood, increases circulation, and makes muscles stronger. But after surgery on the intestines, it's very important to be careful when exercising and follow the instructions given by medical experts. Start with light exercises like walking or stretching, and slowly increase the volume and length of your workouts as your body can handle it. Do not do any tasks that are too hard or that put stress on your abdominal muscles until your surgeon or doctor tells you it is okay to do so. Including a range of exercises, such as aerobics, strength training, and flexibility work, can help you get fitter generally and recover faster. Remember to pay attention to your body and slow down or stop if you feel pain or soreness. You can make a custom exercise plan that fits your needs and limitations by talking to a physical therapist or rehabilitation expert.

Techniques for Dealing with Stress

Getting better after surgery on your intestines can be hard on your emotions. You may feel anxious, frustrated, or depressed during this time. Improving mental health and speeding up the mending process require learning how to deal with stress healthily. Deep breathing, meditation, and progressive muscle relaxation are all activities that can help you relax and feel less stressed.

Doing things that make you happy and fulfilled, like hobbies, spending time with loved ones, or being artistic, can also help you forget about the things that are stressful about recovery. Also, getting help from mental health professionals, support groups, or internet forums can be very helpful for getting emotional support and learning how to deal with tough situations. Putting yourself first and taking care of your mental and emotional health are important parts of holistic healing.

Getting in touch with helpful communities

It can feel lonely to go through recovery, but connecting with supportive groups can give you a lot of help, support, and friendship.

Find support groups or online sites for people who have recently had surgery on their intestines.

 There, you can share your experiences, get advice, and get support from people who know what you're going through. Talking to other people who have been through the same things can give you comfort, validation, and useful tips for handling different parts of your recovery. Including loved ones in your healing process also makes you feel like you belong and builds your support network.

Tell your family and friends the truth about your needs and limits so they can help you and give you emotional support as needed. As you go through recovery, you can celebrate your success, get past problems, and build up your strength and sense of control.

holistic recovery practices take a multifaceted approach to healing after intestinal surgery, looking at the physical, emotional, and social parts of health.

Moving around and exercising safely, learning how to deal with stress, and making connections with supportive communities can help people recover faster and stay healthy in the long run. As you start your path to healing and renewal, don't forget to talk to medical pros, pay attention to your body, and put self-care first.

CHAPTER 9
<u>RECIPES FOR HEALING</u>

Recovery from surgery is an important part of getting better, especially for people who are having surgery on their intestines. The digestive system is very sensitive and needs extra care to help it heal and get better as quickly as possible. Sticking to a healthy, well-balanced diet that supports the body's healing needs is an important part of getting better. In this detailed guide, we'll talk about why a post-surgery diet is important for people who have had intestinal surgery, the nutrients they need to heal, and give you a variety of healing recipes, meal plans, and expert tips to help you stay healthy in the long run.

Rich in nutrients, soups, and broths

Soups and broths that are high in nutrients are important parts of a post-surgery healing diet, especially for people who are having surgery on their intestines.

These liquids are easy to stomach and help the healing process by providing necessary nutrients, water, and warmth. One of the best things about soups and broths is that they give important nutrients in a way that is easy on the digestive system. This makes them perfect for people who may have trouble digesting solid foods right after surgery.

It's important to use ingredients that are high in vitamins, minerals, and protein when making soups and broths that will help you heal from surgery. Bone soup is a popular choice because it has a lot of collagen, which helps tissues heal and is good for your gut. Incorporating veggies like celery, carrots, and leafy greens into the broth also adds important vitamins and antioxidants, making it even healthier.

Besides standard bone broth, plant-based options like vegetable broth or miso soup can also help people who have had surgery on their intestines feel better. People who follow a vegetarian or vegan diet or who may have to follow certain food restrictions because of a medical condition will benefit the most from these choices.

Smoothies and shakes that help the body heal are great for people who have had surgery on their intestines because they make it easy to get nutrients in a liquid form. Because these drinks can be changed to fit different patients' dietary needs and tastes, they are good for a lot of different patients.

When making smoothies and shakes to help with recovery after surgery, it's important to use items that are easy on the digestive system while still giving you a lot of nutrients. Adding fruits like bananas, berries, and mangoes not only makes it taste sweeter, but it also gives you fiber, vitamins, and minerals that your body needs. Green leafy vegetables like spinach or kale can also be added to these drinks to make them healthier. They contain vitamins and phytonutrients that help the body heal.

Protein sources like Greek yogurt, protein powder, or nut butter can be added to smoothies and shakes to help people who need more protein to help repair tissues and muscles. These high-protein foods help you feel full and build muscle while giving your body the important amino acids it needs to heal.

Healthy Main Courses and Sides

Healthy main dishes and sides are very important for helping people recover from intestine surgery because they give the body the nutrients and energy it needs to heal. When making meals for people who have recently had surgery, it's important to include a variety of lean proteins, healthy fats, complex carbs, and fiber-rich foods to help them heal and stay healthy.

Adding lean proteins to meals, like grilled chicken, fish, tofu, or lentils, gives your body the amino acids it needs to repair tissues and muscles.

Adding healthy fats from foods like avocado, nuts, seeds, and olive oil also helps control inflammation and absorb nutrients, which speeds up the healing process even more.

When choosing side items to go with main courses, choosing nutrient-dense foods like quinoa, brown rice, roasted vegetables, or sweet potatoes can help you get more vitamins, minerals, and fiber. Not only are these healthy foods good for you, but they also make you feel satisfied and full, which can help you control your hunger while you're recovering.

Comfort foods like desserts and snacks

Desserts and snacks that make you feel good can be part of a post-surgery recovery diet in small amounts. They can give you pleasure and support your general health. When choosing desserts and snacks for people who have had intestinal surgery, it's important to choose foods that are high in nutrients and easy to digest. Avoid foods that are highly processed or high in sugar, as these can make inflammation or digestive pain worse.

You have more control over the nutritional content and quality of the items when you make your desserts with healthy foods like fruits, nuts, seeds, and whole grains. For instance, making fruit crisps or oatmeal cookies with little extra sugar is a tasty treat that also gives you important vitamins, minerals, and fiber to help your body heal.

Along with treats, eating healthy snacks like Greek yogurt with honey and almonds, hummus with raw vegetables, or homemade trail mix can help you feel full and energized between meals. These snacks have the right amount of carbs, protein, and healthy fats to keep blood sugar levels steady and keep you from losing energy during the day.

 a healthy, well-balanced diet is very important for helping people who have had intestine surgery recover.

People can give their bodies the nutrients and energy they need to heal, reduce inflammation, and stay healthy in the long run by focusing on nutrient-dense soups and broths, healing smoothies, and shakes, nourishing main dishes and sides, and comforting desserts and snacks.

You can also get personalised advice and support from a healthcare worker or registered dietitian to help you recover more quickly after surgery and make it easier to switch to a healthy, long-term eating plan.

CHAPTER 10
KEEPS YOUR HEALTH IN THE LONG TERM

When someone has surgery on their intestines, they usually need to watch what they eat while they are recovering. A well-planned diet after surgery is very important for speeding up recovery, avoiding complications, and maintaining good health in the long run. This complete guide is meant to help you stay healthy in the long run by giving you advice on how to eat well after having surgery on your intestines.

Changing to a diet after recovery:

A very important part of the healing process is switching from a diet after surgery to a diet for long-term health. At first, the focus may have been on foods that were easy to digest to keep the digestive system from getting too stressed and help it heal. As the healing process goes on, though, it's important to slowly add back in a wider range of foods while still focusing on the ones that help with healing and general health.

Focusing on whole, nutrient-dense foods that are high in vitamins, minerals, and antioxidants is one of the most important things to remember when switching to a new diet after healing.

Fruits, veggies, whole grains, lean proteins, and healthy fats are some of these. Eating a variety of foods makes sure that the body gets all the nutrients it needs for a speedy recovery and good health in the long run.

When switching to a diet after healing, it's also important to pay attention to how much you eat and how often you eat. Pay attention to your body's signals for when it's hungry and when it's full, and eat regular, well-balanced meals to keep your energy up and help it heal. Also, drinking enough water is important for digestion, nutrient absorption, and general health.

Even though you may be focused on getting better after surgery on your intestines right now, it's important to think of dietary changes as part of a long-term plan for health and fitness.

Changing your eating habits, getting regular exercise, dealing with stress, and making sure you get enough sleep are all habits that can help you stay healthy for life.

Focusing on small, long-lasting changes instead of big, short-term fixes is one way to build habits that will help you stay healthy for life. Some things that could help with this are slowly eating more fruits and veggies, trying out new healthy recipes, and finding fun ways to stay active.

Also, getting help from doctors, registered dietitians, or support groups can be very helpful when making changes to your food and staying motivated for long-term health. These tools can help people stay on track with their health goals by giving them personalised advice, useful tips, and support.

People who have had surgery on their intestines can get professional help, but many other resources can help them stay healthy in the long run.

Online communities, support groups, and educational materials can help you stay healthy after recovery by giving you knowledge, support, and ideas from other people who have been through the same thing.

Also, using healing recipes and meal plans that are made to fit the dietary needs of people who have recently had surgery can make food preparation easier and help people get the nutrients they need to heal and recover.

These sources often have recipes that are tasty, easy to digest, and full of nutrients. This makes it easier to stick to a diet after recovery while still having tasty meals.

 staying healthy after surgery on the intestines takes a complete plan for nutrition, lifestyle choices, and ongoing support. After recovery, people can improve their general health and speed up their recovery by switching to a diet full of whole, nutrient-dense foods, making healthy habits that will last a lifetime, and using resources for ongoing support.

CONCLUSION

The best way to heal from surgery on the intestines is to take a multifaceted approach that includes medical care as well as nutrition and lifestyle choices. This guide has talked about many different aspects of surgery recovery, from knowing the procedures and what they mean to getting ready for the road ahead.

Because nutrition is so important, we've talked about the basics of a healthy diet, focusing on foods that are high in nutrients, staying hydrated, and getting the right amount of macronutrients. Planning meals has been emphasized as an important part, and sample plans have been given to help people through the different stages of recovery while still making sure they get a range of tastes.

During healing, digestive problems are common. We've given you ways to deal with pain and improve digestive function by eating mindfully and giving your immune system support.

For general health, holistic recovery practices like exercise, managing stress, and getting help from others in the community have also been emphasized.

Healing recipes show how important it is to feed your body nutrient-dense foods, like soups and desserts that make you feel better, which will help you get better and stay healthy in the long run.

As people move on to life after recovery, the focus shifts to maintaining long-term health by building habits and using ongoing support tools.

By following these rules and habits, people can speed up their recovery and build a basis for future health that goes beyond surgery.